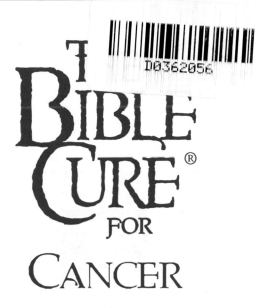

THE
BIBLE
CURE®
FOR
CANCER

DON COLBERT, M.D.

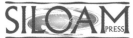

Living in Health—Body, Mind and Spirit

THE BIBLE CURE FOR CANCER
by Don Colbert, M.D.
Published by Siloam Press
A part of Strang Communications Company
600 Rinehart Road
Lake Mary, Florida 32746
www.siloampress.com

Unless otherwise noted, all Scripture quotations are from Holy Bible, New Living Translation, copyright © 1996. Tyndale House Publishers, Inc. Wheaton, Illinois 60189.

Scripture quotations marked KJV are from the King James Version of the Bible.

Library of Congress Catalog Card Number:
99-74595

International Standard Book Number:
0-88419-625-9

01 02 03 04   9 8 7 6
Printed in the United States of America

This War
Is Winnable

Welcome to this investigation of cancer and how to win the fight against it. Does your loved one have cancer? Are you battling this disease in your own body? Perhaps you are simply seeking to avoid cancer in the future. No matter what your circumstances, never forget that cancer is not bigger than God—you can win! The Bible says, "Nothing is impossible with God." You may, at this very moment, be in the greatest battle of your life—but I believe that it will be your greatest victory.

Your first victory over cancer is on the battlefield of fear. I encourage you to make a bold decision to stand up against this Goliath and reach beyond fear to discover hope and faith.

The path to victory is clearer and straighter than ever before. Modern medicine, along with new alternative therapies, all built upon good nutrition and sound principles of daily living, make the experience of cancer much less scary than it once was. Add to this a bold Christian faith to lay hold of the promises of God in Scripture, and you have all you need to arm you against this Goliath of fear and equip you to face any physical or spiritual onslaught. After all, the Word of God says:

> Praise the LORD, I tell myself, and never forget the good things he does for me. He forgives all my sins and heals all my diseases.
>
> —PSALM 103:2–3

I have personally witnessed many people who have fought this battle against cancer and triumphed. This war is winnable, and many others have already won.

Nevertheless, realize that your body is at war every day. Around you and within you are innumerable cancer-causing agents introduced into your body through the air you breathe, the food you eat and the fluids you drink. The information in this booklet will show you what to do about these things, focusing especially upon health-inducing nutrition. God has provided both natural and supernatural agents to battle cancer and help you win the war. Because of all this, you have nothing to fear. "God has not given us a spirit of fear and timidity, but of power, love, and self-discipline" (2 Tim. 1:7).

My friend, this Bible Cure booklet is written to give you great hope. I know it will also help you keep your body fit and healthy for preventing and battling cancer. In these pages, you will

uncover God's divine plan of health
for body, soul and spirit
through modern medicine, good nutrition
and the medicinal power
of Scripture and prayer.

Even if you've already suffered devastation at the hand of cancer, it's not too late to strengthen your faith in God and look to Him more fervently for the peace and healing you need. Throughout this booklet you'll find key scriptures to help you focus on the healing power of God. These inspiring texts will guide your prayers and direct your thoughts toward God's plan of divine health for you in battling cancer or preventing it altogether. You'll discover how to wage the war in the following chapters:

It is my prayer that these practical suggestions for health, nutrition and fitness will bring a new wholeness to your life. May they deepen your fellowship with God and strengthen your ability to worship and serve Him.

—DON COLBERT, M.D.

A Bible Cure Prayer
FOR YOU

Jesus, I thank You that You died on the cross to deliver me from fear and to overcome the power of sickness and death. I thank You that Your name is above every name, and the power of cancer is broken in my life and the lives of my loved ones. Lord Jesus, touch my body at this moment with Your healing power. Cleanse my mind from fear and my body from disease. Give me wisdom to live a healthy life that brings honor to You for the wonderful Creator that You are.

In the mighty name of Jesus Christ, according to the Word of God, I declare that in Christ I have victory over cancer. The power of this disease is broken.

I pray in the name above every name, Jesus Christ, the great Healer. Amen.

Chapter 1

Dare to Take
a Closer Look

Eleanor Roosevelt said, "I gain strength, courage and confidence by every experience in which I must stop and look fear in the face." It's easy to fear the devastating effects of cancer. But we must look it in the face if we wish to defeat it. We can begin to fight cancer by first seeking to know the enemy a little better. So let's start by finding out just how much cancer exists, why it happens and what first steps we can take to overcome it.

How Much Cancer?

How prevalent is the diagnosis of cancer today? Studies have shown that one out of every three Americans will develop cancer and one out of six people diagnosed with cancer will die as a result.

1

Cancer is truly a widespread killer.

Cancer Is Losing the Battle

At first glance these statistics may appear frightening. However, the truth is that the battle against cancer is already being won. The number of cancer deaths in the nation has decreased steadily over the past decade because of increasing knowledge about this disease and great advances in medicine.

In addition to the powerful breakthroughs experienced in the medical arena, miracles by the healing touch of God happen every day. Instantaneous miracles are performed in a moment by the power of the Holy Spirit. I have seen many people whose triumph over cancer, even in its advanced stages, can only be described as miraculous. And I know other medical doctors who would agree that they too have also witnessed such dramatic occurrences.

I have also witnessed numerous other healings that take place over a longer period of time. These patients pray, trust God's Word and use natural therapies that include good nutrition, supplements, herbs and vitamins. This approach provides an arsenal of weapons to battle the many factors that cause cancer.

What Are the Contributing Factors?

The more rapidly growing cancers are usually made up of very immature cells. Each normal, healthy cell has a specialized function that it is designed and "destined" to perform. Consider a small child. He or she

> *He personally carried away our sins in his own body on the cross so we can be dead to sin and live for what is right. You have been healed by his wounds!*
> —1 Peter 2:24

may grow up and become a businessman, a doctor, an engineer or an attorney. Yet another young child with the same apparent destiny—in terms of having good parents and a good environment—may grow up and, instead of performing a meaningful job, may become a gang member, a murderer, a bank robber or a serial killer. Something happened in this individual's life to change his destiny. Instead of becoming a productive citizen, he became a criminal.

Likewise, cancer cells are simply immature cells that, instead of growing up to perform their

proper function, remain immature. In this unde-
veloped form, the cells feed on the body, stealing
nutrition from the body in order to grow larger
and larger. They grow up into killer cells.

What causes these cancer cells to grow out of
control? And why do some people develop cancer
when others do not? Some of the answers involve
the strength of an individual's natural defenses
against the unnatural growth of cells, how an individual keeps his or her body strong for the battle
and how many and what kinds of cancer-produc-
ing agents a person's body is forced to fight.

It's a proven fact that approximately 70 to 80
percent of cancers are caused by the food we eat,
the air we breathe and the water we drink, as well
as lifestyle and environmental factors. All of these
things have a cumulative effect over a person's life
span. Let's look at these factors a little more closely,
grouped under three key threats to our healthy
cells:

Threat #1: Our diet. About one-third of all
cancer deaths occurring in our nation each year
are due to dietary factors, with another third
due to the use of tobacco. In a sense, this is encouraging, because here is where we can make
a huge difference in the spread of cancer—

simply by making changes in our lifestyles.

Remember that something is constantly being done about the attacks on your healthy cells. Every minute of every day it's happening. While you are working, walking, eating and relaxing, your body is already winning a silent war that is raging around and within you. It's because of your amazing immune system. This system, along with your blood cells and vital organs, is wonderfully designed by God to overcome even the most powerful attacks by cancer-causing agents in foods and the environment. Be thankful that this wonderful system is always at work to protect you.

So how can we strengthen our immune systems and keep them strong? Our diets directly impact our immune systems, either positively or negatively. Since our immune systems are our bodies' first and strongest line of defense against cancer, we must be diligent to care for them and to strengthen them by eating the right foods and avoiding harmful foods. What you eat makes all the difference!

All of this will become clearer as you continue reading this book. For now, simply note that the ancient Hebrew texts of the Bible reveal guidelines for eating that can lower your risk of cancer.

Consider the avoidance of animal fats, for example. The Bible declares:

> You must never eat any fat or blood. This is a permanent law for you and all your descendants, wherever they may live.
> —LEVITICUS 3:17

The fat referred to in these passages comes from the portions of meat containing the most dangerous substances: low-density lipoproteins, or LDL. As you'll see, Scripture also suggests that natural foods provide the best nutrition for our bodies. Problems in the average American's diet occur when daily meals ignore biblical guidelines and consist of:

- Excessive animal fats, including heavy oils
- Excessive sugar, which weakens the immune system and actually fuels the growth of cancer (which is fed by sugar)
- Devitalized foods, including salt, white flour, processed foods, cured meats and margarine
- Toxins in our food, such as nitrites and food additives

- Heavy metals, such as the mercury sometimes found in fish

Threat #2: Our environment. God has created healthy substances that not only give us natural energy but also help prevent disease. But people have created environmental toxins that wear down the body's ability to resist cancer, things such as solvents, pesticides and heavy-metal residues.

These toxins can build up in our bodies and damage our DNA, the molecular building blocks of life, causing originally healthy cells to grow out of control. City air is one of the biggest offenders. It's often contaminated by hydrocarbons, smog, cigarette smoke and other toxic substances. In rural areas, about two billion pounds of pesticides, many of which are carcinogenic, are sprayed on American crops each year. Our farm animals feed on millions of pounds of antibiotics and hormones as well.

Billions of pounds of poisonous garbage sit rotting in toxic waste sites, and over fifty thousand of these sites in America threaten to seep their toxins into the water supply. As a result of chemicals like DDT, abnormalities can be found in the eggshells of many birds and in the reproductive organs of many animals. Fortunately, DDT has been banned since 1973 because of its widespread effects on wildlife, yet other chemicals have taken its place.[1]

In spite of growing concern about toxins in our environment, many of our city water supplies contain chlorine, aluminum, pesticides and many other toxins. If we were to focus on the effects of chlorine alone, we could become quite alarmed. For when chlorine reacts with other organic materials, it forms carcinogens (cancer-causing agents) associated with colon, rectal and bladder cancers.

> *But he was wounded and crushed for our sins. He was beaten that we might have peace. He was whipped, and we were healed!*
> —Isaiah 53:5

Threat #3: Our free-radical reactions. Certain toxins are extremely damaging to human DNA, which is the genetic blueprint for the life of the body's cells. These toxins from the environment can trigger free-radical reactions in our cells. To understand these reactions, consider the oxidation process. Burn wood in a fireplace, and smoke is a by-product. Likewise, when you metabolize food into energy, oxygen oxidizes (or burns) the food in order to produce energy. This process does not create smoke like burning wood in a fireplace, but it does produce dangerous by-products known as free radicals. These are molecules that have set electrons roaming free to cause damage in other cells.

Free radicals, considered a kind of molecular shrapnel, can damage cells and start chain reactions within the body. They can damage the DNA and in some cases can cause cells to mutate, forming cancerous growths. Amazingly,

> *Pay attention, my child, to what I say. Listen carefully. Don't lose sight of my words. Let them penetrate deep within your heart, for they bring life and radiant health to anyone who discovers their meaning.*
> —PROVERBS 4:20–22

scientists have discovered that each cell in the human body undergoes between one and ten thousand free radical hits to the cell's DNA every day. But if our bodies lack a strong antioxidant defense system, then our systems become increasingly susceptible to damaged DNA and therefore to cancer.

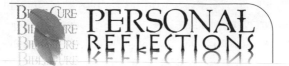
Threatening the Threats

The "threats" we've been looking at are not the last word on our health. As Christians, we have the Lord at our side, making sure that nothing brings us ultimate defeat—not even death itself. Here is how the apostle Paul put it:

> If God is for us, who can ever be against us? Since God did not spare even his own Son but gave him up for us all, won't God, who gave us Christ, also give us everything else?
>
> —ROMANS 8:31–32

Take a moment right now to consider your level of faith in this promise as it relates to your battle with cancer.

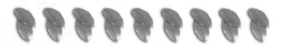

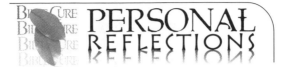

PERSONAL REFLECTIONS

DEAR GOD, I believe. Please help my un-belief in the following ways:

_____

_____

_____

_____

_____

_____

_____

_____

_____

_____

_____

Thank You, Lord! Amen.

What's a
Person to Do?

As cancer-causing agents increase all around us, we can follow God-given strategies to win the war against their harmful effects. Thankfully, God has provided for us both natural methods and supernatural power to overcome. So don't quit. Don't give up. Don't surrender to fear. Cancer is not the last word—God's Word is!

Always remember that you aren't helpless against cancer. You can begin now to take some practical, positive steps toward defeating it. Just start implementing my suggested "prescriptions" in each chapter. (However, since I cannot give you all the answers for your unique situation, always consult a physician to determine the prevention or treatment plan that's best for you.)

The great gospel singer Pearl Bailey once said, "People see God every day; they just don't recognize Him." In your battle with cancer, look for God in everything around you. Recognize His presence in all you do, for He cares for you with a love that runs deeper than the oceans.

God is our refuge and strength, always ready to help in times of trouble. So we will not fear, even if earthquakes come and the mountains crumble into the sea.

—PSALM 46:1–2

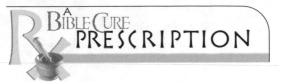

Take Some First Steps

Ready to take some first steps in fighting cancer?
Here's a summary list of some practical things you
can start doing right now. Check the ones you'd
like to begin today:

- ❑ I'll begin reevaluating my diet and think-
  ing about healthier eating habits.

- ❑ I'll limit my high-fat foods, especially from
  high-fat meats.

- ❑ I'll avoid cigarette smoke, and I will determine to never smoke or quit if I do smoke.

- ❑ I'll take time to read and memorize God's
  Word.

- ❑ I'll determine to choose faith and reject
  fear, because God's Word says Jesus Christ
  defeated cancer and disease.

Chapter 2

Power Up
With Power Foods

What a powerful person is our Lord Jesus Christ! Along with all His power, the thing I like to consider is the deep compassion He uses in exercising His power. Read through the Gospels and you'll see Jesus going from place to place, constantly offering healing and forgiveness to all who approached Him. One of my favorite accounts is this story of healing from a truly dreaded disease:

> Large crowds followed Jesus as he came down the mountainside. Suddenly, a man with leprosy approached Jesus. He knelt before him, worshipping. "Lord," the man asked, "if you want to, you can make

me well again." Jesus touched him. "I want to," he said. "Be healed!" And instantly the leprosy disappeared.

—MATTHEW 8:1–3

Healing people is still Jesus' desire today. Have you approached Him lately for His healing? For His compassion? For His power?

Jesus is ready to give you all these good things. And in this brief chapter, I want to assure you that the Lord has already with great compassion built into our foods a good amount of power, too—healing and cancer-fighting power!

Your Food—
and Divine Power

Yes, it's true. We already have access to certain "power foods" that can give our bodies tremendous defenses against cancer. These power-food weapons are tremendous defenses against cancer. These power-food weapons are called phytonutrients. How good are they? Just imagine being able to drink milkshakes that could lower cholesterol, eat burgers that could help fight cancer and cheesecakes that could cool menopausal hot flashes and mood swings. Well,

16

God's ideal food sources for all of this exist in His created order, and science is just beginning to discover them.

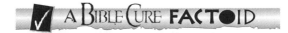

Exciting, isn't it? You'd probably like to know more about the numerous power-food sources of the phytonutritients you need to live healthy and fight disease. We'll start with those isoflavones mentioned above.

Your Phytonutrients and the Soy Connection

Iso what?

Yes, I know it's another strange term. But you're getting used to them by now, right? Isoflavones are natural estrogens found in soybeans and soy products. Since researchers at the National Cancer Institute have reported marvelous cancer-fighting properties in these chemicals, I heartily recommend them to you. Here is where you can get yours from soy foods providing a range of 30 to 50 milligrams per serving:

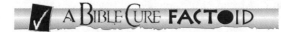

A BIBLE CURE FACTOID

Places to Get Your Isoflavones

Roasted soy nuts (1 ounce)
Soy flour (½ cup)
Soy grits (¼ cup)
Textured soy protein (½ cup, cooked)
Yellow, green vegetables or
black soybeans (½ cup, cooked)
Regular soy milk (1 cup)
Tempeh (½ cup)
Tofu (½ cup)

But do these foods really do battle in the cancer war? Through clinical findings, we know that

Japanese women have one-fourth the amount of breast cancer as American women, and Japanese men have one-fourth the risk of prostate cancer as American men. Why are breast and prostate cancer so much lower among the Japanese than Americans? Soy products! The Japanese consume approximately thirty times more soy products than Americans do.[2]

To understand how soy foods do their amazing work, you need to know that cancers create new blood vessels so they can continue to grow and nourish their out-of-control cells. It's a process called angiogenesis. The potent phytonutrients in soy often block the formation of these new blood vessels and, as a result, starve the tumors!

> *One day while Jesus was teaching, some Pharisees and teachers of religious law were sitting nearby. (It seemed that these men showed up from every village in all Galilee and Judea, as well as from Jerusalem.) And the Lord's healing power was strongly with Jesus.*
> —Luke 5:17

Here's how it works in greater detail: Soy contains phytoestrogens, which are phytonutrients that are only one one-thousandth as strong as estrogen. However, they tend to block the estrogen receptors in our cells, which then decrease the tumor-promoting effect of high estrogen levels. So, soy's phytoestrogens actually inhibit the ability of cancer cells to reproduce themselves and grow into tumors.

These benefits aren't just limited to women. For the men, there is aromatase, an enzyme in a man's body that converts testosterone to estrogen. A 1989 study of eight thousand Hawaiian men found that those who ate the most tofu had the lowest occurrences of prostate cancer.[3]

See why I firmly believe that everyone should eat some type of soy food on a daily basis? There are different sources of soy, of course. You could start by trying soy milk, tofu, miso soup, soy protein extracts, soy yogurt, soy flour or even isoflavone tablets (which can be taken as a substitute). But I think the easiest way to obtain your soy on a daily basis is to drink a soy protein milkshake that you can mix by adding a frozen banana to some flaxseed oil, and even some soy milk. For a real treat, try a soy fruit smoothie:

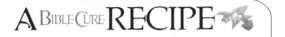

A BIBLE CURE RECIPE

MAKE YOURSELF A
SOY FRUIT SMOOTHIE

2 cups vanilla-flavored soy beverage, well chilled
1 cup frozen sliced peaches
1 medium banana, cut into chunks
8 medium strawberries
¼ teaspoon ground cinnamon

In a blender, combine the soy beverage, peaches, bananas, strawberries and cinnamon. Blend until smooth and creamy.

Makes 2 servings.[4]

A Few Other Lifesavers

I want to remind you to keep praying and seeking God as you make these dietary changes! Take a lesson from the prophet:

> When I had lost all hope, I turned my thoughts once more to the LORD.
> —JONAH 2:7

Even if you don't feel like praying, keep on approaching the throne of grace every day; your prayers do come before the Lord. I know it can be difficult. If you have some form of cancer, the pain and weakness can bring on bouts of discouragement.

Those who wrote the Bible learned about God in the same ways that you and I learn about Him. They became discouraged and fearful at times too. David wrote:

> *Then if my people who are called by my name will humble themselves and pray and seek my face and turn from their wicked ways, I will hear from heaven and will forgive their sins and heal their land.*
> —2 CHRONICLES 7:14

> The righteous cry, and the LORD heareth, and delivereth them out of all their troubles. The LORD is nigh unto them that are of a broken heart; and saveth such as be of a contrite spirit. Many are the afflictions of the righteous: but the LORD delivereth him out of them all.
> —PSALM 34:17–19, KJV

22

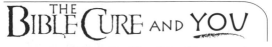

BIBLE CURE AND YOU

What Do You Need?

The promise of Scripture is clear when it comes to praying for what we need. This applies to all our circumstances, even when we face cancer and seek healing. Listen to the words of Jesus: "I tell you, keep on asking, and you will be given what you ask for. Keep on looking, and you will find. Keep on knocking, and the door will be opened. For everyone who asks, receives" (Luke 11:9–10). Think about what you need most in order to apply these words to your life these days. Mark the lines below with the specific letter(s) denoting your particular need:

I= I need more INFORMATION about health and/or insight into God's will.

C= I need more COURAGE to face my enemy, cancer.

W= I need more WILLPOWER so I can be self-disciplined and make good choices.

F= I need more FAITH in order to believe God's promises and persevere in my trials.

___ When you hear about new treatments, medicines and therapies

___ When your doctor says you need chemo-therapy

___ When you feel impatient with God's timing

___ When you've experienced another health setback

___ When you're depressed because of the stress and pain of cancer

___ When you must relocate to a new place for health reasons

___ When you worry that you might get sick (or sicker)

___ When you can't eat the things you want

___ When you have to make lifestyle changes because of sickness

___ Other: _____

- Think: *What things help me the most when I'm discouraged in my battle with cancer? What first steps can I take, right now, to pursue at least one of those things?*

I'm simply saying: Keep implementing the changes in your diet that make for good health, and keep trusting in the Lord's goodness toward you in all things. Now, with that said, I'll quickly recommend another group of foods containing potent phytonutrients: the cruciferous vegetables. These wonderful vegetables include:

- Broccoli
- Cabbage
- Brussels sprouts
- Cauliflower

Cruciferous vegetables, like soy, provide numerous different phytonutrient compounds, including indoles. Indoles are able to convert estrogen from a cancer-promoting form into a cancer-preventing form. They do this by converting estradiol to estrone, which also results in a reduced incidence of breast cancer.

If you hate the taste of cruciferous vegetables, broccoli capsules are now available; you can take them once or twice a day. Or take "indole-carbinol-phytonutrient" capsules, which are available at health food stores or through ordering on the Internet (www.livinghealthier.com).

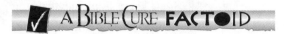

Food Sources for Your Phytonutrients

Phytonutrient	Food Source	Benefits to Your Health
Lycopene	(Tomatoes)	Antioxidant cancer prevention heart protection
Sulphoraphane	(Broccoli)	Cancer prevention and cell detoxification
Polyphenol	(Green Tea)	Cancer prevention antibacterial detoxification
Organo-Sulphur	(Garlic)	Immune system enhancement
Flavonoids	(Onions, Apples)	Heart protection cancer prevention
Resveratrols	(Red Wine)	Prevents PGE_2 formation
Ellagic Acid	(Strawberries, Grapes, Walnuts)	Anticancer properties

One more thing to know: Foods such as wheat grass, alfalfa, barley grass, spirulina, chlorella and blue-green algae are all extremely high in chlorophyll. Chlorophyll has been found to have anticancer effects, since it protects the DNA from damaging radiation. These foods have also been shown to have antiviral, antitumor and anti-inflammatory properties. In effect, such foods can actually inhibit carcinogens in cooked meats and even in cigarette smoke. I recommend that patients make a chlorophyll drink containing each of these potent power foods. Here's how:

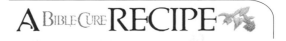

A BIBLE CURE RECIPE

DR. COLBERT'S DAILY MILKSHAKE

Take a teaspoon of each of these powders and blend in a mixer with orange juice. Blend until smooth and creamy.

- Alfalfa
- Wheat grass
- Barley grass
- Spirulina
- Chlorella
- Blue-green algae

Drink this mixture on a daily basis.

I personally drink the concoction above, along with freshly squeezed orange juice, as soon as I wake up in the morning. I also take it in the evening as soon as I get home from work. But what about you? Will you give some of these things a try?

My dear friend, I know you may feel a bit beaten up by cancer at the moment. That is certainly natural and easy to understand. Is there a brokenness in your spirit as well? Perhaps there's even a feeling of hopelessness settling in. Take heart! I offer you these encouraging words to conclude this chapter:

> *Don't worry about anything; instead, pray about everything. Tell God what you need, and thank him for all he has done.*
> —PHILIPPIANS 4:6

> God uses broken things. It takes broken soil to produce a crop, broken clouds to give rain, broken grain to give bread, broken bread to give strength. It is the broken alabaster box that gives forth perfume . . . it is Peter, weeping bitterly, who returns to greater power than ever.
> —VANCE HAVNER

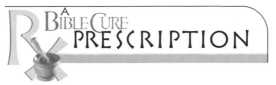

Choosing Your Power Foods

Are you eating your power foods? From the list below, check the ones you eat regularly and circle those you need to start eating NOW!

Broccoli	Cabbage	Brussels sprouts
Cauliflower	Tomatoes	Garlic
Green tea	Apples	Wheat grass
Alfalfa	Barley grass	Spirulina
Chlorella	Blue-green algae	Maitake mushrooms
Red Olives	Strawberries	Raspberries
Grapes	Walnuts	Black currants

Chapter 3

Healthy Fats?

Imagine sinking your teeth into a nice, juicy, inch-thick steak. As you savor that bite, you butter your potato, throw on a mound of sour cream and then dig in again. Later, you follow it all with a luscious ice cream sundae, whipped cream piled high. What could be better?

Actually, it's not so great not for your health, anyway. To stay healthy you'll have to cut back on the steak and ice cream.

And a few other things, too . . .

No Surprise, Right?

Of course, none of this is news to you. You've no doubt heard, time and again, about the dangers of high-fat, high-sugar, high-sodium diets when it comes to your overall health. But did you know that certain diets are linked to an increased incidence of cancer? This is especially true for the high-fat diet, which is strongly related to colon, rectal and prostate cancers. There's real hope here, though, because you can definitely reduce the risk of cancer by sticking to a diet that includes high proportions of fruits, vegetables, grains and beans while limiting the amounts of red meats, dairy products and other high-fat foods. The Bible clearly recommends this way of eating:

> Look! I have given you the seed-bearing plants throughout the earth and all the fruit trees for your food.
> —GENESIS 1:29

When we eat the kind of diet the Creator of our bodies intended, we naturally build a strong immune system that defends against cancer. Here's how it happens: We know that hormone-like compounds (prostaglandins) greatly affect our immune systems. (When most people hear the word *hormone,* they think of sex hormones, such as estrogen. However, the human body has hundreds of hormones that regulate everything from thyroid function to blood sugar levels.) Many different forms of prostaglandins exist; some are beneficial, and some are extremely detrimental.

PGE_2 is a bad one. It may sound a little like *Star Wars,* but PGE_2 is not a robot. It's a dangerous prostaglandin linked to the formation of prostate,

> *O Lord, you alone can heal me; you alone can save. My praises are for you alone!*
> —JEREMIAH 17:14

colon and breast cancers. The intake of too much polyunsaturated fat, such as safflower oil, corn oil and sunflower oil will cause an increase of PGE_2. A high level of PGE_2 can then increase our risk of these forms of cancer. Also, eating insufficient amounts of fish oils, flaxseed oil and essential fatty acids like omega-3 will also cause an increase of PGE_2. Conversely, extremely low-fat or no-fat diets tend to increase the PGE_2 in our bodies, too. That's why the right balance of essential fatty acids is so crucial.

Essentially Acidified?

Essential fatty acids (EFAs) like omega-3 cannot be manufactured in the body and must be consumed either through diet or supplements. EFAs help the body repair and create new cells. Omega-3, in particular, is also apparently effective in limiting the spread of cancer.

> A very new finding is that the omega-3 fatty acids can actually create special roadblocks in the body, making it harder for cancer cells to migrate from a primary tumor and start new colonies. Cancers that spread (metastasize) are the real killers.[1]

Clearly, EFAs like omega-3 are incredibly beneficial. Here are some omega-3 foods to include in your diet as a way to help prevent and battle cancer: raw nuts (walnuts), flaxseeds and flaxseed oil, fish, (salmon, mackerel, halibut, tuna, herring and cod) and fish oil. Obviously, it's important to know which fats to eat and which ones to avoid when it comes to preventing those harmful prostaglandins I mentioned above.

Enjoy Those Good Fats

In my desire to keep things simple and practical for you, I'm going to focus on just one fantastic source of good fat to pursue in your nutritional plan. It's the humble olive with its beautiful, golden oil.

Believe it or not, olives can help you fight cancer. The fat found in olives is an excellent, healthy substance that our bodies need. The diet of biblical times included an abundance of olive oil and other Mediterranean foods that promote health and healing. God described the Promised Land for His people as being a place that included the nutritious olive:

> *The Spirit of the Lord is upon me, for he has appointed me to preach Good News to the poor. He has sent me to proclaim that captives will be released, that the blind will see, that the downtrodden will be freed from their oppressors, and that the time of the Lord's favor has come.*
> —LUKE 4:18–19

> For the LORD your God is bringing you into a good land of flowing streams and pools of water, with springs that gush forth in the valleys and hills. It is a land of wheat and barley, of grapevines, fig trees, pomegranates, olives, and honey.
> —DEUTERONOMY 8:7–8

Olives and olive oil contain a substance called *squalene,* which has anticarcinogenic effects. In our day, Greek women have only one-third the incidence of breast cancer as American women. Yet approximately 40 percent of the Greek's caloric intake is from fat.[2] However, most of their intake of fat comes from olive oil. Because of these facts, I recommend cooking with extra-virgin olive oil whenever you have to stir-fry.

In fact, whenever a recipe calls for adding any type of oil, why not use extra-virgin olive oil? Also, when you sit down to eat a salad, choose a dressing with an extra-virgin olive oil base, and remember to add plenty of olives to your salad and other dishes. It's commonly known that people on a Mediterranean diet, which contains large amounts of olive oil and olives, have a decreased risk of breast cancer.

> *And no doubt you know that God anointed Jesus of Nazareth with the Holy Spirit and with power. Then Jesus went around doing good and healing all who were oppressed by the Devil, for God was with him.*
> —ACTS 10:38

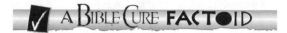

God's Mediterranean Health Food

Olive Oil
Three basic types of olive oil work great for cooking and for pouring on salads or on pasta:

Extra-virgin olive oil: I recommend using this kind of olive oil whenever possible. It's usually the purest and most tasty. Look at the color. The deeper the color, the more intense the olive flavor. This type of olive oil has the most disease-fighting substances.

Pure or virgin olive oil: It's paler than extra-virgin and is usually used for frying in low to medium heat.

Light olive oil: This is often used for its healthy benefits to the heart, having the mono-unsaturated fats without the strong olive taste. It's good for high-temperature frying.

Avoid the Bad Fats

I've mentioned bad fats, but how do we recognize them? Usually they're labeled as saturated and polyunsaturated. Since they are associated with many different kinds of cancer, learn to recognize these dangerous kinds of fats and avoid them.

Polyunsaturated fats reside primarily in safflower oil, sunflower oil and corn oil. Saturated fats come from animal products such as whole milk, red meat, pork, skins of chicken and turkey, bacon, luncheon meats, cheese, ice cream and butter. Stay away from them as much as possible.

In particular, avoid margarine. Does that come as a surprise to you? I believe that transfats are the most dangerous form of fats. These are man-made fats, created by hydrogenating vegetable oil. The process involves heating the oil to a high temperature and then bubbling hydrogen gas into it, causing the liquid vegetable oil to harden and become a man-made food called *margarine*. Unfortunately, margarine is added to most of our baked goods, breads, pastries and many of our processed foods. Hydrogenated fats not only increase the risk of heart disease, but also will increase the risk of cancer. So if you've just got to spread one

> *Jesus traveled throughout Galilee teaching in the synagogues, preaching everywhere the Good News about the Kingdom. And he healed people who had every kind of sickness and disease.*
> —MATTHEW 4:23

or the other on your toast, choose a little butter over margarine.

Long ago, God told the people of Israel:

> If you will listen carefully to the voice of the LORD your God and do what is right in his sight, obeying his commands and laws, then I will not make you suffer the diseases I sent on the Egyptians; for I am the LORD who heals you.
>
> —EXODUS 15:26

This promise is for us, too. He is still the Lord who heals us today. And I believe He still calls us to listen carefully to His voice and to do what is right. That must be our approach when it comes to all aspects of living, including how we eat.

> *And this same God who takes care of me will supply all your needs from his glorious riches, which have been given to us in Christ Jesus.*
> —PHILIPPIANS 4:19

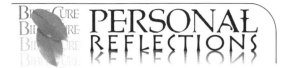
How Does It Apply?

Think about how Exodus 15:26 applies to you today. Have you considered lately what it means for you to follow God's leading and to do the right thing? Complete the sentences below, and then jot a brief prayer to the Lord in light of your responses.

- I know that I am hearing God's voice when . . .
- The last time this happened, I responded by . . .
- It's hardest for me to do what is right when . . .

Dear God,
Thank You for . . .

_____ .

Please help me to . . .

_____ .

Amen.

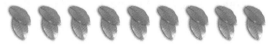

Do This for a Fatter
Chance at Health . . .

I'll close this chapter with just two simple words of advice about your fat intake:

First, eat fish. Remember that the healthiest fats you can eat are the omega-3 fatty acids, which come primarily from cold-water fish such as salmon, mackerel, tuna, halibut and cod. (These other omega-3 foods have a protective effect against cancer: flaxseed oil, cod liver oil, dark green vegetables, broccoli, kale, collards, Swiss chard.) One significant study in Europe found that lower cancer rates were associated with higher fish and fish oil consumption, whereas higher cancer rates apparently came with increased animal fat consumption.[3]

My second word of advice is to double dose with flaxseed oil every day. This oil is extremely high in the omega-3 fatty acid called alpha-linolenic acid. Freshly ground flaxseeds contain a type of fiber called lignan, which also has anti-cancer effects. It acts similarly to soy in inhibiting the enzyme that converts testosterone or other hormones into estrogen. I personally take one tablespoon of flaxseed oil twice a day. In addition, I grind five teaspoons of flaxseed in a coffee grinder at least once a day.

So, how do you eat ground flaxseed? You can eat it by the spoonful, add ground flaxseed to cereals or put them in a fruit shake. Another easy way to

> *He spoke,*
> *and they were*
> *healed—snatched*
> *from the*
> *door of death.*
> *—PSALM 107:20*

get flaxseed into your diet is to add ground flaxseed to the ground meal of muffins, breads and other baked goods. You can replace a few tablespoons of flour in your recipes with ground flaxseed without noticeably changing the taste or texture of your baked goods. (Note: Do not cook with flaxseed oil. It oxidizes and forms a very dangerous fat. I also throw the bottle out after it's been used for a month, since the oil is very prone to oxidation after the bottle has been opened.)

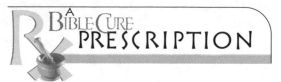

R **A BIBLE CURE PRESCRIPTION**

Cooking Healthy

List three ways you will include olive oil in your food preparation:

1. _____

2. _____

3. _____

Describe how will you use flaxseed in your baked goods:

_____

_____

_____

_____

_____

Circle the days of the week on which you will eat fish:

Mon   Tue   Wed   Thu   Fri   Sat   Sun

Chapter 4

Winning With Fiber and Supplements

I f you want to win the war against cancer, you'll need to eat the things that battle it. I'm going to fill this chapter with lists of these things, so you can have no doubt about what to do. As you consider each one, please don't become overwhelmed. Take one step at a time. Add the good things you are missing, and let go of the others that have become harmfully habitual. Soon you'll realize that your eating habits have been transformed.

> Have compassion on me, LORD, for I am weak. Heal me, LORD, for my body is in agony.
>
> —PSALM 6:2

If this is your plea also, remember that God

hears and answers. He also invites you to change for the better with His help, and He is clearly on your side. Now, let's begin those lists . . .

Get Your Fiber-Fill!

Listen to those folks on TV telling you about your fiber needs. They're right! Fiber is extremely important in preventing cancer because it binds and helps the body excrete cancer-causing chemicals. For example, studies have concluded that diets high in fiber actually lower the risk of breast cancer. In Finland, people consume a diet that is both high in fat and high in fiber. However, the incidence of breast cancer is quite a bit lower there than in other industrialized countries like the U.S., where people eat a a lot of fat but consume little fiber.[1]

A high-fiber diet will also decrease estrogen by binding it so that it can be passed out of the body. It increases the bulk in the stool, which speeds up elimination, thereby minimizing the amount of time toxins are able to stay in contact with the wall of the colon. One form of fiber found in the cell walls of citrus fruits is a very potent cancer fighter called modified citrus pectin. This substance may inhibit disease by preventing cancer cells from adhering to tissue. Modified citrus pectin, along with soy products, is excellent in preventing the metastatic spread of cancers.

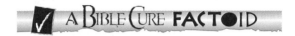

A BIBLE CURE FACTOID

Seven Basic Sources for Fiber in Your Diet

I recommend rotating the sources I've listed below, since each has its own function in helping your body prevent cancer, especially colon cancer. Always take fiber products separately from other medications or supplements, which can lessen the effectiveness of the fiber. The seven sources are:

- Bran
- Cellulose—outer layers of vegetables and fruits
- Gum—guar gum
- Hemicellulose—apples, bananas, corn, beans, beets, peppers, whole-bran cereals
- Lignin—Brazil nuts, carrots, green beans, peas, peaches, potatoes, strawberries, potatoes
- Mucilages—chickweed, comfrey, mullein, flaxseed, okra
- Pectin—apples, cabbage, okra, carrots, beets

The many different forms of fiber include psyllium, oat bran, rice bran, ground flaxseeds, modified citrus pectin and others. Find your favorite form of fiber, and take it on a daily basis. I personally prefer fresh ground flaxseeds. However, you may use over-the-counter psyllium products such as PerDiem Fiber, Metamucil or oat bran. Now let's look at how to fight the war against cancer by using these supplements: amino acids, vitamins, minerals and herbs.

Add This Amino Acid

Throughout this booklet, we have identified wonderful substances that God has created for our health and disease prevention. Glutamine is one of the most remarkable of all. It's the most abundant amino acid, found in muscle tissue, blood and spinal fluid. It is also the only amino acid that easily passes through the blood into the brain. Glutamine, a powerful antioxidant, is extremely important to immune system function because it increases natural killer cell activity. It also inhibits

> *I will give you back your health and heal your wounds, says the Lord.*
> —JEREMIAH 30:17

the harmful prostaglandin PGE_2. I recommend taking approximately 1000 milligrams of L–glutamine thirty minutes before each meal.

Glutamine supplements are available through health food stores, though you can get it by eating certain raw plants, such as spinach and parsley. It should not be taken by persons with cirrhosis of the liver, kidney problems, Reye's syndrome or any type of disorder that can result in an accumulation of ammonia in the blood. Be certain to consult with a physician before taking this or any other supplement.

Take Your Vitamins, Dear . . .

Mom was always reminding us, so let's take heed! Certain vitamins are extremely important for immune system function and cancer prevention. Here's your list of what to take:

- *Vitamin A*—approximately 5,000 International Units a day
- *Beta carotene*—approximately 25,000 International Units a day
- *Vitamin C*—500 to 1000 milligrams, two to three times a day
- *Folic acid*—800 to 1000 micrograms a

day. It may be the most important B vitamin in the prevention of cancer. It is very important for the repair of DNA. Patients consuming the highest amounts of folic acid had a significant reduction in the risk of developing premalignant polyps of the colon.[2] Take this vitamin daily to boost immune activity and assure necessary DNA repair.

- *Vitamin E*—at least 400 International Units per day. Vitamin E protects the thymus gland, which is one of the main glands responsible for immune function. It has also been shown to decrease the rate of prostate cancer by as much as 32 percent. Other studies have linked a high intake of vitamin E to decreased risk of both breast and uterine cancer. I recommend at least 400 International Units of vitamin E a day. It is best to get all four forms of vitamin E, including alpha, beta, gamma and delta tocopherols, which are found in Unique E. You can find most of these vitamins in a comprehensive multivitamin formula. At the end of this book, we provide information on obtaining Divine Health Multivitamins.

Mind Your Minerals, Too

Certain minerals are critical for your immune function. Both *zinc* and *selenium* are extremely important for strong immune functioning. Unfortunately, much of the soil in the U.S. is deficient in selenium. People with a low intake of selenium have an increased risk of developing cancers, especially cancers of the stomach and the esophagus. Some of the highest incidences of stomach cancer are found in China, in areas where the selenium levels are lowest in the soils.[3] Strive to consume at least 200 micrograms of selenium per day.

Calcium is another mineral that may prevent cancer from developing. It is especially important in preventing colon cancer. Calcium can bind to very toxic acids and help remove them from the body. This decreases the amount of toxins exposed to the lining of the colon. You may get calcium from low-fat skim milk and skim-milk

> *As the sun went down that evening, people throughout the village brought sick family members to Jesus. No matter what their diseases were, the touch of his hand healed every one.*
> —LUKE 4:40

cheese, or you may consume calcium supplements (approximately 1,000 milligrams a day for pre-menopausal women, and 1,500 per day for post-menopausal women).

IP$_6$, known as inositol hexaphosphate, has strong antitumor functions. It may be able to cause cancer cells to mature and behave in a way that is similar to normal cells. IP$_6$ is also able to strengthen our immunity and boost the activity of our natural killer cells. This powerful antioxidant comes from whole-grain cereals, legumes and soybean seeds. It resides in the bran layer of rice and wheat seeds. In corn, it is found in the germ portion of the kernel.

Finally, *shark cartilage* has also been shown to be beneficial in both preventing and treating cancer. It apparently inhibits angiogenesis, both in test-tube conditions and in living organisms.

Heal With Herbs

Certain herbs have potent anticancer effects. *Rosemary* prevents formation of the dangerous prostaglandin PGE$_2$ and promotes the phase two detoxification enzymes in the liver. Rosemary has also been shown to prevent cancer-causing chemicals from binding to the DNA in cells, thus inhibiting tumors.

Another important herb is *curcumin*, which prevents formation of the dangerous prostaglandin PGE_2. It blocks the formation of cancers at all stages of development. Take 300 milligrams of curcumin per day, or for an even greater effect, take it three times a day.

Milk thistle is another potent herb, also known as silymarin, which we've mentioned previously. Take milk thistle at a dose of 175 milligrams, two times a day.

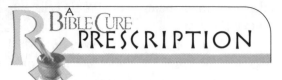

Fighting Cancer With Fiber

Daily, I will get my fiber from (list at least 5 ways):

1. _____

2. _____

3. _____

4. _____

5. _____

The supplements I will take are:

_____

_____

The herbs I will eat are:

_____

_____

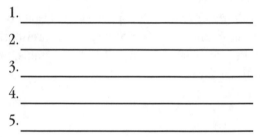

Chapter 5

Determine
to Detox!

When the great King David experienced healing from the hand of God, he lifted his heart in praise, declaring, "O LORD my God, I cried out to you for help, and you restored my health" (Ps. 30:2). I hope that you too are lifting your heart daily to the Lord. Yes, crying out to Him for help whenever you need it. You don't even have to use words, for as Victor Hugo once said, "Certain thoughts are prayers. There are moments when, whatever be the attitude of the body, the soul is on its knees."

As you seek the Lord in your thoughts and prayers, remember that the restoration of health, from a medical point of view, usually involves some kind of detoxification of the body to make way for the restoration of healthy processes. So let's delve into the detoxification process in this chapter. It's such an important part of your body's cancer-fighting arsenal, and you can learn to support and strengthen it.

Taking Out the Trash

Just as you take the trash out to your front curb every Wednesday morning (or is it Friday?), so your body must remove the various wastes and impurities from its system. This isn't just a weekly event, though; it's happening all the time, primarily through the work of your liver.

The liver is our most important body organ for detoxifying all the harmful chemicals we take in on a daily basis. It detoxifies harmful substances such as pesticides, food additives and pollutants, among other things. So be sure to maintain your liver's health to help you win the war against cancer. Damage to your liver can result from drinking alcohol, being overweight, abusing drugs or chemicals or eating an improper diet.

Along with detoxification, the liver has important functions in body metabolism, such as aiding in digestion and energy production. As the body digests proteins (and through the bacterial fermentation of food in the intestines), ammonia is produced. Along with other toxic substances in the body, ammonia is combined with less toxic substances in the liver and then removed through the kidneys.

The point is, without the liver detoxifying our bodies, we would be filled with toxins like ammonia, metabolic waste products, insecticide residues and other harmful chemicals. So we depend heavily on our livers for good health. This powerful cleansing organ has an amazing two-phase system of neutralizing and eliminating toxins from the body. It does this by employing various detoxification enzymes. Here's how the process works:

Phase one: First, many of the toxins passing through the liver are made water-soluble. But in doing so, many may actually become more active,

> *Wherever he went—in villages and cities and out on the farms—they laid the sick in the market plazas and streets. The sick begged him to let them at least touch the fringe of his robe, and all who touched it were healed.*
> —Mark 6:56

thus becoming more damaging. There are as many as a hundred different enzymes involved in the phase one system of detoxification.

Phase two: While phase one breaks the toxins down by making them more water-soluble, phase two attaches special detoxifying enzymes to the toxins. This process of attaching the toxins with a detoxifying enzyme is called conjugation, and the timing must be synchronized with phase one.

The substance that supports these enzymes and detoxifies the body is called glutathione. It is the most abundant antioxidant in our bodies, manufactured from whey protein, glutamine, n-acetyl-cysteine and cruciferous vegetables among other things. Glutathione also recycles antioxidants such as vitamins C and E, and it is extremely important in immune system function.

Now that my technical explanations are complete, I want to stop here and ask you: Wouldn't you agree that we could benefit from knowing what kinds of nutrients and chemicals help the detoxifying processes? I can't refer to all of them in this little booklet. But let's consider two of the most critical substances that you can begin putting into your diet right away.

Getting Enough
Milk Thistle

Milk thistle is a wonder of God's creation. Also called wild artichoke or Mary thistle, it is a unique flavonoid and antioxidant containing potent liver-protecting substances (it even stimulates the production of new liver cells). The active ingredient in milk thistle is silymarin.

The nice thing about milk thistle is that you can take it as a capsule. If you're using it to address problems of alcohol-related liver problems, hepatitis, cancer or cirrhosis, take 200 milligrams three times daily (total 600 milligrams).

You must give it at least eight weeks before determining its usefulness for you. If you are taking it to detoxify or as a preventive, about 175 milligrams twice daily will suffice.

Along with milk thistle, some other foods that stimulate phase two detoxification include broccoli, spinach, cruciferous vegetables, green tea, turmeric tea, Brussels sprouts, strawberries, raspberries and grapes.

Adding Sufficient Zinc

Zinc is an essential mineral found in oysters,

crabmeat, beef, liver, eggs, poultry, brewer's yeast and whole-wheat bread, among other sources. It maintains taste and smell acuity, normal growth and sexual development, and it is important for fetal growth and the healing of wounds. Its main importance to liver function is this: It protects the liver from chemical damage. After all, with all the garbage that passes through your liver every day, it needs some help to keep itself healthy.

One way the liver suffers is through heavy-metal toxicity in our bodies, especially toxicity from mercury. Are you wondering if you have this problem? The following is a list of symptoms related to mercury toxicity. Test yourself for these symptoms, and if you score high, I recommend that you consult your doctor. High levels of mercury in your body can interfere with enzyme activity and can eventually result in blindness and paralysis.

Heavy metals in the body can produce the following symptoms:

- Depression
- Dizziness
- Gum disease
- Insomnia
- Muscle weakness
- Dermatitis
- Fatigue
- Hair loss
- Memory loss
- Excessive salivation

If you think this kind of toxicity may be the case for you, you would need to detoxify your body of mercury by taking in high-chlorophyll foods (such as chlorella) and by supplementing with zinc. Zinc deficiency has been associated with many different cancers, including prostate, esophageal and lung cancers. I recommend taking approximately 30 milligrams of zinc a day. (Note: Be cautious with zinc consumption. If you take both iron and zinc, do so at different times, since they interfere with each other. Also, taking zinc at higher doses can depress the immune system.)

Now, a final word about detoxification. Remember that we are whole persons, more than mere bodies. Because of this, we are called to stay pure in our minds and spirits,

> *A vast crowd was there as he stepped from the boat, and he had compassion on them and healed their sick.*
> —MATTHEW 14:14

too. How can we do it without meditating on our Creator and His Word day and night? I have spoken of the trash so marvelously cleansed from our bodies by liver function. But the Scriptures also speak of a cleansing of heart and soul.

Let this be a comfort to you! It is the Lord who cleans us up inside, because we have no power to do it ourselves. That's good news; when the Great Physician comes in and detoxifies us, He does a perfect job.

> Purify me from my sins, and I will be clean; wash me, and I will be whiter than snow.
>
> —PSALM 51:7

> But if we confess our sins to him, he is faithful and just to forgive us and to cleanse us from every wrong.
>
> —1 JOHN 1:9

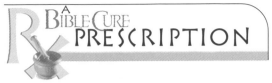

Protecting Your Liver

Check the things you will do to protect your liver in preventing cancer:

❑ Take milk thistle.

❑ Eat broccoli, spinach, cruciferous vegetables, green tea, turmeric tea, Brussels sprouts, strawberries, raspberries and grapes.

❑ Avoid excessive consumption of alcohol.

❑ Avoid foods and liquids containing environmental toxins such as pesticides and heavy metals.

Chapter 6

Antioxidants
to the Rescue

L ook out! A fire just flared in your kitchen!
What do you do?

If you've got an extinguisher nearby, you'd be
silly not to reach for it. Anything to put out the
flame would certainly come in handy.

But what fights the fire of rapidly multiplying
body cells, the potential cancers that may eventually rage out of control?

Extinguish Those Free Radicals!

God's Bible cure in winning the battle against cancer includes a powerful fire extinguisher in our
food antioxidants. They're amazing substances that
help prevent the oxidation that produces free radicals in our bodies. Now a free radical is not a

terrorist trying to firebomb our embassy; rather, it's a defective molecule spraying molecular shrapnel that damages our cells. This certainly isn't what God wants to be happening in our bodies.

> Dear friend, I am praying that all is well
> with you and that your body is as healthy
> as I know your soul is.
>
> —3 JOHN 2

Free radicals are the enemies of a prospering body. Remember that we compared them to the smoke released by a fire. They are molecules that have lost an electron, and they will steal an electron (oxidation) from another compound, making that compound unstable. As a result of this chemical reaction, vital cell parts sustain damage. Some estimates calculate that the cells in our bodies take up to ten thousand hits from free radicals each day.

God's wonder agents, the antioxidants, help prevent cancer by blocking and repairing free radical reactions. Simply stated, an *antioxidant* is a vitamin, mineral, enzyme, phytonutrient (plant nutrient) or food that has the ability to bind free radicals and neutralize them. How does it do this? The antioxidant pairs with the electron of the cell that is spinning out of orbit. In that way, it stops a dangerous chain reaction—the beginning of the mutation of a cell that can eventually lead to the formation of cancerous growths. Let's look a little more closely at some of the key antioxidants that you can reach for right now:

Grape seed or pine bark. Powerful anti-oxidants called proan-thocyanidins include pine bark extract (which is pycnogenol)

> *Kind words are like honey—sweet to the soul and healthy for the body.*
> —PROVERBS 16:24

and grape seed extract. Grape seed and pine bark extract are twenty times more potent than vitamin C and fifty times more potent than vitamin E as scavengers of free radicals. These antioxidants are also quite effective in maintaining a healthy level of the structural protein collagen, which holds our cells together.

Collagen is like a glue that keeps our skin from sagging and aging. I recommend that you take 50 to 100 milligrams of grape seed or pine bark, or both, daily. Grape seed oil, in particular, has wonderful benefits. It contains no cholesterol or sodium and has a light, nutty taste that really brings out the taste in foods. It's great for cooking. Remember to buy only the cold-pressed variety that has no preservatives.

Lipoic acid. This antioxidant is both fat-soluble and water-soluble. It helps to recycle other antioxidants, including vitamin C and vitamin E, thus extending their antioxidizing functions. Although researchers have done hundreds of studies (covering over forty years) revealing how lipoic acid energizes metabolism, there is still great excitement about this vitamin-like substance. Many recent studies focus on how it improves the physique, combats free radicals, protects our genetic material, slows aging and helps protect against heart disease and cancer.[1]

There simply isn't enough alpha-lipoic acid in our bodies, so I'd recommend 50 to 100 milligrams a day as a preventive measure against diseases caused by free-radical attacks. I routinely place diabetics on much higher doses of up to 300 milligrams, two to three times a day.

Coenzyme Q_{10}. Here's another potent antioxidant that is not only very beneficial to the heart but also has a strong impact on the immune system and may prevent cancer. I recommend at least 50 milligrams a day as a preventive measure, and I routinely place cancer patients on 200 to 300 milligrams a day.

Lycopene. Another potent antioxidant, lycopene resides in the red pigment in pink grapefruits, watermelons and tomatoes. A study with health professionals involving forty-seven thousand patients revealed a significant reduction in prostate cancer associated with high levels of lycopene; seven thousand patients revealed a significant reduction in prostate cancer associated with high levels of lycopene-rich food consumption. Most of the lycopene intake came from tomatoes: sauce, juice, paste and pizza topping.

Studies also revealed that men who ate ten or more servings of these tomato foods per week had a 45 percent less risk of prostate cancer than those who did not eat this way.

> *Then you will gain renewed health and vitality.*
> —PROVERBS 3:8

Yellow fruits and vegetables. Phytonutrients are antioxidants that come from plants, and they are some of the most potent anticancer compounds in existence. You can easily add them to your diet through eating certain fruits and vegetables, as listed below. Other potent phytonutrients are carotenoids, found in yellow and orange fruits and vegetables. These vegetables are full of alpha and beta carotene and lutein, which is available in high concentrations in spinach, kale and collard greens. They protect against cancer, especially breast cancer. Try to eat some of these daily: carrots, sweet potatoes, pumpkin, cantaloupe, corn and yellow squash.

Start With the Lowly Carrot

I know my numerous recommendations can seem overwhelming at first, so I'll suggest one simple starting point for your daily antioxidant intake. Just begin eating more of one of God's truly remarkable creations: the carrot. Research has demonstrated that the beta carotene in carrots helps us with night vision, lowers cholesterol and helps us battle both heart disease and cancer.

Do you have a juicer? Probably the best way to get the highest dose of carotenoids is to drink a half to a full cup of fresh carrot juice daily. I do this on a daily basis in the midmorning. Get out your juicer. Processing carrots in a juicer makes a perfect carrot cocktail. The juicer breaks apart the carrot's fibers, releasing the beta carotene.

As you drink your tasty, free-radical extinguishing snack, keep in mind this encouraging research regarding beta carotene. In a study of 1,556 middle-age men, researchers from the University of Texas School of Public Health in Houston, as well as two medical centers in Chicago, found that those with the highest levels of beta carotene and vitamin C in their diets had a 37 percent lower risk of death from cancer than the men with the lowest levels of beta carotene.[2]

Now that is good news! And here's another bit of good news straight from God's Word. I leave it with you as you consider where to buy that next bag of carrots . . .

> Don't be afraid, for I am with you. Do not be dismayed, for I am your God. I will strengthen you. I will help you. I will uphold you with my victorious right hand.
> —Isaiah 41:10

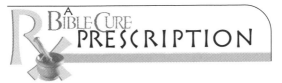

Assembling Your Antioxidant
Weapons Against Cancer

Now you're ready to load up your arsenal against cancer with powerful foods and supplements that contain antioxidants. Evaluate how well you are doing now and determine to increase your intake of antioxidants in the coming weeks. Put an "x" on the line where you are now and "✔" on the line what you want to do in the days ahead.

Eating carrots:

    1 __ 2 __ 3 __ 4 __ 5 __ 6 __ 7 __ 8 __
Never   Sometimes   Often

Consuming foods containing lycopene:

    1 __ 2 __ 3 __ 4 __ 5 __ 6 __ 7 __ 8 __
Never   Sometimes   Often

Circle the foods you will begin eating more often:

sweet potatoes   pumpkins   yellow squash
   cantaloupe   corn   tomatoes
 pink grapefruit   watermelons

Check which supplement you plan to add to your daily intake:

❑ Grape seed or pine bark   ❑ Lipoic acid
❑ Coenzyme Q_{10}

Chapter 7

Take a Soul Check—and a Walk

S omeone once said that the best way out is always through. It's true in your fight against cancer. By combining God's natural substances with His positive prescriptions for the mind, emotions and spirit, you can build a powerful immune system. No toxin will be able to get a foothold in your body, and fear will gain no place in your mind.

The Bible cure offers a bold, fearless response to meet the challenge of cancer. That response is faith in the powerful promises of God's living Word.

Take Five Now

We've talked about taking various foods and supplements throughout this booklet. These focus on strengthening and protecting your physical body.

But what do you take for the mind and spirit—two of the other parts of you that greatly affect your overall well being? Consider these suggestions:

Take refuge in the Scriptures. God's Word breaks the destructive power of certain deadly emotions, such as fear, rage, hatred, resentment, bitterness and shame. I encourage you to quote scriptures related to them at least three times a day, on a continuous basis. Also read and meditate on Bible passages like 1 Corinthians 13, the chapter on love, since there is no greater force in the universe than the power of God's love. It is able to break the bondage of any destructive emotion.

Take up positive attitudes. Related to Scripture reading is the practice of putting on the positive, healthy emotions that it speaks of—love, joy, peace, patience, kindness, goodness and self-control. We know that certain emotions are associated with lowered immune function and higher cortisol levels. Approaching life with the biblical attitude prescription will help you avoid the damaging effects of stress, fear and worry. Several decades ago, S. I. McMillen, author of the best-selling *None of These Diseases,* confirmed what I'm saying:

> Peace does not come in capsules! This is regrettable because medical science recognizes that emotions such as fear, sorrow, envy, resentment, and hatred are responsible for the majority of our sicknesses. Estimates vary from 60 percent to nearly 100 percent.[1]

Take time to offer a blessing. Naturally, I recommend that everyone bless their food prior to eating it. I believe this will cover us with a certain degree of protection, even if we eat the wrong types of food. Of course, do avoid the habit of eating the wrong types of foods! However, remember that we are NOT perfect, and we are not under the Law, but under grace. We will, at times, slip up.

Take some daily exercise. How often do you exercise during the week? Did you know that getting out and jogging, walking or bicycling—or participating in any type of regular, moderate form of exertion—can help you avoid cancer? It's time to get up off that couch and get active! Regular exercise is one of the best ways to maintain good health. Besides, I have a feeling that God takes pleasure in the health of our bodies:

> He gives power to those who are tired
> and worn out; he offers strength to the
> weak . . . Those who wait on the Lord will
> find new strength. They will fly high on
> wings like eagles. They will run and not
> grow weary. They will walk and not faint.
> —Isaiah 40:29, 31

According to the American Medical Association, people who exercise regularly have lower incidences of cancer in general. The great thing about exercise is that it makes our digested food move more quickly through the colon. That way, it can't sit there and ferment, causing potentially cancer-causing irritations. Exercise also lowers the risks of endometrial and breast cancers by reducing a woman's body fat (which produces estrogen, a facilitator in the growth of some cancers).[2]

The best form of exercise is aerobic exercise, which includes brisk walking, cycling, swimming or jogging.

> *He forgives all my*
> *sins and heals all*
> *my diseases.*
> —Psalm 103:3

Some doctors say that just thirty minutes of exercise every other day can reduce the risk of breast cancer by 75 percent! You see, cancer cells are anaerobic, which means they don't thrive in high-oxygen environments. Exercise pumps oxygen to your cells, giving your body added ability to win the war against cancer.

Take a laughter break. Some of us hardly ever laugh. But we need to do so often. In fact, one of the best ways to prevent cancer is to laugh. The Book of Proverbs says, "A cheerful heart is good medicine, but a broken spirit saps a person's strength" (17:22). Excessive stress is quite dangerous because it increases our cortisol levels, which then suppresses the immune system. When the immune system is suppressed, cancerous cells can begin to form and grow.

Although there's no question that environment and genes play a significant role in our vulnerability to cancer and other diseases,

> *A cheerful heart is good medicine, but a broken spirit saps a person's strength.*
> —PROVERBS 17:22

the emotional environment we create within our bodies can activate mechanisms of destruction or repair.[3]

It's true; our emotions work like medicines— good medicine or bad. And laughter really is the best medicine! Watching funny movies, going to comedy clubs where there is good clean humor, telling jokes and simply enjoying life is the best prescription for stimulating the immune system. Comedian George Burns was a hundred years old when he passed away. He abused his body for most of those hundred years by smoking, drinking and carousing. It may be because he had a joyful heart, though, that he was able to live so long despite a toxic diet of alcohol, cigars and bad food.

Take Courage—for Tomorrow

In addition to focusing on all the nutritional steps you can take to battle cancer, it's essential to maintain a merry heart. As you've seen, the war against cancer is by no means a hopeless effort. Just stay curious about the things you can do to prevent it. Pursue those things; make those changes; remain joyful in the love of God. I have no doubt that if you do this, God's great promise will be true of you:

> Yes, your healing will come quickly. Your godliness will lead you forward, and the glory of the LORD will protect you from behind.
>
> —ISAIAH 58:8

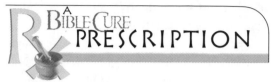

Your Soul Check

What are three passages of Scripture that have impacted your life as you read this booklet?:

1. _____

2. _____

3. _____

Name three positive attitude characteristics that you want God to develop further in your life.

_____

_____

_____

What forms of exercise will you commit to pursue regularly from today forward?

_____

_____

Conclusion

The most important ingredient in your Bible Cure prescription is faith in a God of incomprehensible power, might and love. God's power is already at work in your body at this very moment breathing life into your heart, mind and spirit—for there is no life outside of Him. God's healing power is at work in your body right now healing every cut and scratch—for no healing takes place apart from God's Spirit. Greater still is the power of God's love to reach into the depth of your need at this very moment in response to your faith. God loves you beyond anything you could ever imagine. If you have cancer, ask Him—at this very moment—to touch you, to help you and to heal you.

—Don Colbert, M.D.

Notes

CHAPTER 1
DARE TO TAKE A CLOSER LOOK

1. Dr. Karl N. Harrison, "DDT: A Banned Insecticide." Article published by the University of Oxford Web site based in the Chemistry IT Center, Department of Chemistry, 1999.

CHAPTER 2
POWER UP WITH POWER FOODS

1. Jean Anderson and Barbara Deskins, *The Nutrition Bible* (New York: William Morrow and Co., 1995), 319.
2. For further information about breast cancer, see the November 1994 issue of the *Medical Sciences Bulletin,* published by Pharmaceutical Information Associates, Ltd.
3. Severson, "A prospective study of demographics, diet, and prostate cancer among men of Japanese ancestry in Hawaii," *Cancer Res, Vol. 49,* (1989), 1857.
4. Selene Yeager, *New Foods for Healing* (Emmaus, PA: Rodale Press, 1998), 495.

CHAPTER 3
HEALTHY FATS?

1. Clara Felix, *All About Omega-3 Oils* (Garden City, NY: Avery Publishing, 1998), 32.
2. A. Trichopoulou, K. Katsouyanni, S. Stuver, D. Trichopoulos, L. Tzala, C. Gnardellis, E. Rimm, "Consumption

of Olive Oil and Specific Food Groups in Relation to Breast Cancer Risk in Greece," *Journal of the National Cancer Institute,* 87: 110–116, January 18, 1995.

3. C. Caygill, A. Charlett, M. Hill, "Fat, fish, fish oil and cancer," *Journal:* Br J Cancer 1996; 74(1):159–64. C.

Chapter 4
Winning With Fiber and Supplements

1. H. N. Englyst et al., "Non-starch Polysaccharide Concentrations in Four Scandinavian Populations," *Nutrition & Cancer* 4:50–60, 1982.

2. "Multivitamin Use, Folate, and Colon Cancer in Women in the Nurses' Health Study" (full text) *Annals of Internal Medicine,* 1 October 1998. 129:517–524.

3. L. C. Clark, The epidemiology of selenium and cancer. *Fed Proc* 1985; 44:25842590. Also note: L. C. Clark, K. P. Cantor, W. H. Allaway, "Selenium in forage crops and cancer mortality in U.S. counties," *Arch Environ Health* 1991; 46:37–42. G. N. Schrauzer, D. A. White, C. J. Schneider. Cancer mortality correlation studies III. Statistical associations with dietary selenium intakes. *Bioinorg Chem* 1977; 7:23

Chapter 6
Antioxidants to the Rescue

1. Summarized from Richard A. Passwater, Ph.D., in "Lipoic Acid: The Metabolic Antioxidant."

2. Selene Yeager, *New Foods for Healing* (Emmaus, PA: Rodale Press, 1998), 119ff.

Chapter 7
Take a Soul Check—and a Walk

1. S. I. McMillen, *None of These Diseases* (Westwood, NJ: Revell, 1963), 7.

2. AMA Health Insight, General Health, by Theodore Berland, www.ama-assn.org/Insight/Gen_Hlth/Fitness/Fitnes2.htm: Fitness Basics, Medical Review by Jeffrey Tanji, M.D., University of California, Davis, posted: Nov. 20, 1997.

3. Bernie S. Siegel, *Peace, Love, and Healing* (New York: Harper and Row, 1989), 35.

A Note on Alternative Resources . . .

If you are suffering from cancer and haven't received successful results from conventional cancer hospitals, consider the following alternative cancer medical centers:

Oasis Hospital is a Christian-based hospital in Tijuana, Mexico. Dr. Ernesto Contreras and his son, Dr. Francisco Contreras, are recognized authorities on both conventional and alternative cancer therapies. The toll-free phone number is 888-500-HOPE.

Another excellent hospital for alternative cancer therapy is the American Biologics Hospital in Tijuana, Mexico. The toll-free phone number is 800-227-4473.

Dr. Stanislaw Burzynski in Houston, Texas, uses peptides called antineoplastons, which are partially effective against brain cancer. His phone number is 281-531-6464.

Don Colbert, M.D., was born in Tupelo, Mississippi. He attended Oral Roberts School of Medicine in Tulsa, Oklahoma, where he received a bachelor of science degree in biology in addition to his degree in medicine. Dr. Colbert completed his internship and residency with Florida Hospital in Orlando, Florida. He is board certified in family medicine and has received extensive training in nutritional medicine.

If you would like more
information about natural and
divine healing, or information about
Divine Health Nutritional Products®,
you may contact
Dr. Colbert at:

Dr. Don Colbert

1908 Boothe Circle
Longwood, FL 32750
Telephone: 407 331 7007

Dr. Colbert's website is
www.drcolbert.com.

BIBLE CURE

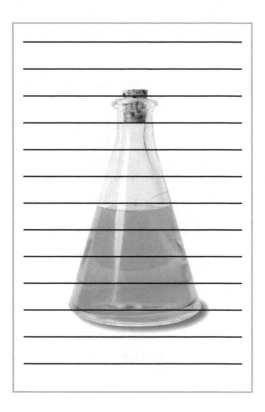

_____
_____
_____
_____
_____
_____
_____
_____
_____
_____
_____
_____
_____

BIBLE CURE

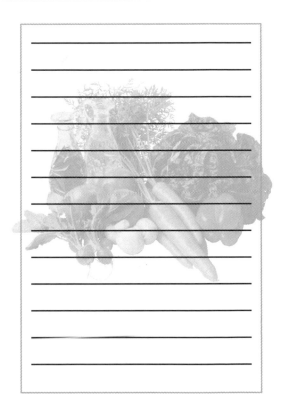

Pick up these other Siloam Press
books by Dr. Colbert:

Walking in Divine Health

What You Don't Know May Be Killing You

The Bible Cure® Booklet Series

SILOAM PRESS

A part of Strang Communications Company
600 Rinehart Road
Lake Mary, FL 34726
(800) 599-5750